D1797615

Beyond Diet Foods:

Best Food For Healthy Eating, Fat Burn, Weight Loss, Optimal Nutrition and Balanced Diet

By

Brittany Samons

Table of Contents

Beyond Diet Foods:

Best Food For Healthy Eating, Fat Burn, Weight Loss,

Optimal Nutrition and Balanced Diet

By Brittany Samons

Introduction

Do you really now your body? Do you know which foods are good for you? Beyond diet is about that, to learn what foods you can or can't eat according to your body type. So what do you need to do first? Well the first step will be finding out what your body type is. And how do you do this? There are some questions that you will have to answer in order to determine it. Once you know which is your body type you will be introduced to the best foods for you. With this you will learn the correct food and liquid portioning in a day. The objective: to lose weight in a healthy way.

Chapter 1. Let's Begin The Process

The Beyond diet was developed based on the principles of eating foods that don't increase glucose levels in blood; it is a gluten-free diet that promotes eating foods with low glycemic index by educating and motivating people while they are dieting. The Beyond diet slogan claims: "Stop counting calories, start eating well and start living!" So why don't give it a chance? It sounds like lots of benefits.

Probably you have been yo-yo dieting for years and you have become tired of the ups and downs, probably other diet programs failed and you have lost your faith in dieting. When dieting you temporarily alters what you normally eat but you don't change eating habits and when you get tired of that diet you return to those bad habits. Diets are "controlled starvation" and starvation leads to a slow metabolism and slow metabolism leads to weight gain. Besides that, when you starve yourself you have other symptoms like hunger and fatigue, so why to continue dieting?

Beyond Diet is a way to change eating habits for life! It is a long-term strategy that offers healthy and delicious food to you. It has a scientific foundation, and you can implement each principle each and every day. You don't have to change all your old habits all of a sudden, just take charge of your health and your weight, one thing at a time will make more sense and you will notice the changes sooner than you expect.

Chapter 2. Change Your Mind

It requires some time getting into the right state of mind to start the new lifestyle habits. People has been bombarded with products campaigns for years so first of all clear your mind of all media information, try to avoid TV commercials and magazines ads from healthy, light, low-fat products (we'll get there later) and start believing that you can change your habits while feeling great. Free yourself from any negative thinking and replace negative thoughts with positive ones. Remember that accomplishment requires work, commitment and dedication but the result worth it.

Everybody knows that it is important to eat healthy and have a well balance diet. Beyond diet restricts certain foods according to your body type but it is very easy to follow once you have change your dieting habits. If you can replace certain foods and have a huge will power you are in the correct path; the Beyond diet is for you! The program is about establishing a lifestyle, not just following a "diet" that people will drop with the time.

So once you have joined the Beyond diet program, you answer the questions then you have the list of foods that best suits your metabolism type, next you will monitor the amount of servings for each meal and the percentage of fat, carbs and protein recommended for you. In other words there are three main steps in the Beyond Diet:

1) Determine your metabolism type

2) Create a personal meal plan

3) Learn which healthy foods work for you

Each person has a unique body's biochemistry that requires certain amounts of proteins, carbohydrates and fats to work optimally. Learning your metabolism type will help you to lose weight without starvation or cravings in a healthy way. You can be a Carb type, a Protein type or a Mixed Type and certain foods are ideal for each metabolism type, just because a food is healthy doesn't mean is healthy for you!

Forget about starving or skipping meals, it is important for you to consume three meals: breakfast, lunch and dinner and two snacks in between. Don't let yourself become extremely hungry because you will crave and wish to eat every food at your sight. The Beyond diet also suggests to drink plenty of water; in fact half of your weight in ounces.

Another advised is to avoid processed foods and better try to eat natural products; organic ones are preferred. You can write down your shopping list and have a trip to the farmer's market! This way you will have all necessary things to prepare your meals. Don't feel overwhelmed you can replace worst calorie foods with healthy substitutes one by one, making small but significance changes it's what matters at first to adjust to this new lifestyle. The most important step toward weight loss is to choose and identify which foods are good for you. There is a very simple rule: If it is natural, I mean if it grows or occurs in nature eat it, if it is artificial then don't. Include in your meals fresh unprocessed fruits and vegetables, unroasted nuts (from trees and ground), whole seeds and grains, unadulterated fats, meat products and dairy, in the other side do not choose packaged food, hydrogenated oils, high fructose corn syrup products (watch out! This is very popular) frozen meals, cookies, cakes, aspartame, sucralose. Chemicals included in processed foods irritate the gastrointestinal system causing bloating, constipation or gas. These toxins are stored in fat cells, more fall cells in your body more toxins you have in it and of course this can lead to many diseases. From now on it is important only to eat clean unprocessed food.

Chapter 3. Metabolism Types

Protein Type: People with protein type metabolism crave rich fatty foods like pizza or sausages and they love food and love to eat! Often feel hungry and simple snacks are not enough for them. For this type of metabolism eaten too many carbs leads to crave sugar and once you start you want more and more obviously lose weight will be more difficult. Eating the wrong food causes fatigue, anxiety and nervousness. A diet high in proteins and fats but low in carbohydrates is the perfect diet for this type of metabolism. It should be a well-balanced diet between various carbs in form of fruits, vegetables and grains and the correct amount of proteins and fats. Protein type metabolizes food faster than the other types (that's why they are always hungry!) so they should choose heavier protein choices like whole eggs, beef or diary. They will need to eat protein at every meal including snacks; this will control blood sugar levels and make them feeling satisfied. It is good for them to eat often, otherwise will suffer from low blood sugar. Bread, crackers and pastas made from wheat are a NO and they should avoid most fruits because these ones converted fast into sugar. The best fruits for this metabolism type are apples and avocadoes. Protein types should eat approximately 45% of proteins, 35% carbs and 20% fats.

Carb Type: Opposite to the protein type, carb type people have weak appetites and they live happy with a minimal amount of food, they don't care too much about food and don't give it too much thought. They frequently skip meals because they have too much work to do each day. These "workaholics" live in "starvation mode" and pass extended periods of time without eating. Most of carb type people are addicted and dependent on caffeinated beverages to help them through the day, this weakness even more their appetites. They have high tolerance for starchy vegetables and baked goods. The perfect diet for them is a diet with more carbohydrates than proteins or fats (they still need protein), white poultry and white fish are good choices, they can tolerate and feel great on a high carbs low fat diet. For this metabolism type will be good to eat high fat proteins occasionally because they can cause depression, fatigue and lethargy. Some people tend to metabolize diaries poorly so if you feel fatigued after eating them it will be better to avoid them. Eat plenty of low starch vegetables like green salads or broccoli, say NO to bread, pasta and grains. Nuts and seeds are a good option for snacks but not for meals. Carb types should eat approximately 20% of protein, 70% carbs and a 10% of fats.

Mixed Type: People with this type of metabolism require an equal balance between proteins, carbs and healthy fats. For them variety is very important in their diets. This type is the easiest of the three because they have many options where they can choose. They can be hungry at meals but not so much in between and they don't suffer cravings (lucky them!) This type must incorporate high fat and low fat proteins, as well as high and low starch carbs. For the mixed type it is important to be familiar with the requirements of the other two types so they can find the perfect balance. Finding the right balance will be the key to succeed and feeling great. Mixed type must eat 40% of protein, 50% of carbs and 10% of fats.

Chapter 4. What to Eat

1) Proteins: There are plenty foods loaded with proteins. Choose lean meat, fresh fish (better than frozen) and poultry. Do not choose microwave dishes they have a big amount of sodium. Nuts, seeds and eggs are also a great option to get protein in a natural way.

2) Drinks: Of course water is the best choice but if you are not so into it you can also drink tea, milk (non-fat) and if you can't leave soda at least drink a low-fat one.

3) Dairy Products: All your dairy products must be low fat; milk, cheese and yogurt. If you don't want dairy you can have coconut or almond milk.

4) Good Carbs: These carbs here are not the enemies they promote fat loss. Eat breads made of quinoa, millet, sprouted grains. A sweet potato is a good option for good carbs and of course fruits and vegetables.

Recommended foods:

1) Spinach

2) Lettuce

3) Asparagus

4) Strawberries

5) Apples

6) Mango

7) Almonds

8) Peanut Butter

9) Organic eggs

10) Raw milk

11) Wild Fish

12) Shrimp

13) Grass-fed beef

14) Free-range chicken

15) Ezekiel bread

16) Quinoa

17) Wild rice

18) Oatmeal

19) Buckwheat

20) Lentils

21) Avocado

22) Raw organic butter

23) Coconut oil

24) Extra-virgin olive oil

25) Unsweetened cocoa

26) Organic red wine

Meat, Poultry and Eggs

Beyond Diet Program recommends to eat organic food, it is more expensive but it worth your health. Have you ever think about the animals you eat? Where did they come from? Animals that become our food should be as healthy as the food it was fed. These animals are fed with low quality grains. Why cows are eating grains? Besides pigs and chicken live in very bad conditions with not enough space and hygiene. That's why organic food is better and expensive.

Yogurt

It is one of the healthiest foods as it contains live cultures that are good bacteria in large amounts. It is healthy as it source (again grass fed cows) and yogurts with added ingredients lose nutritional value. The best way to eat yogurt is to eat it plain, Greek yogurt is a great option. People who are lactose-intolerant can consume it without side effects.

Milk

A recommendation from Beyond Diet program is to drink raw milk from free roaming grass fed cows. Thousands of people consume raw milk and they are even healthier than people who consume pasteurized and homogenized products. It is kind of difficult to get it but it worth it. If you can't get it at least try organic certified, this milk doesn't contain antibiotics, hormones or pesticide residues. If you can't afford organic then substitute it for coconut or almond milk.

Soy

There are many soy products in the market from soy sausages to soymilk, from soy burgers to energy bars. Soy has become a very popular product nowadays with its healthy claims but the truth is that soy is bad for health, Soymilk is worse than cow's milk. Studies have proven that it contains isoflavones (phytoestrogens) that causes several conditions. So take a look at your pantry and discard each product that contains soy protein, soybean and soy oil.

Grains

You probably have eaten a huge amount of carbohydrates in form of bread, potatoes, cereal, baked goods, pasta and rice. The worse thing is that these carbs have been consumed in the form of processed food that leads to heart diseases and obesity. Excess of carbohydrates are stored as fat with severe consequences to health. The key to success in weight loss is to find the right balance in the quantity of carbohydrates consumed every day. So leave grains aside and choose some good carbs like the ones in fruits and vegetables.

Bread

The most popular and consumed carbohydrate around the world is bread and guess what? It is not so good as you think; it leads to poor health and excess weight. If you love bread choose one made from sprouted whole grains, it is the best you can consume. Wheat bread has cheated people for years; it causes constipation and irritable bowel syndrome. If you are intolerant to wheat or gluten it is better to exclude all kinds of bread from your diet.

Water

Most people don't drink the recommended amount of water, they don't understand how important it is and all the benefits it provides to a good health and in the losing weight process. Think about this: our bodies are composed of 75% of water and it should be maintained like that, any variation from the natural balance is wrong. Some of water benefits are:

- It helps the body to metabolize stored fat

- It helps the body to get rid from waste

- It is a natural diuretic and laxative

Is not good to drink cold water, because it will stay in the stomach until warm to body's temperature, the best is to drink it at room temperature. You should drink half of your body weight in ounces each day; if you exercise add some more ounces to prevention dehydration.

Sugar

For every person that consumes five pounds of sugar another eats 295 pounds of it! Processed sugar that is contained in many products is the worst to consume; it can literally be considered poison. Having excess sugar in the body eventually affects every organ in it. Sugar leads to diseases like diabetes; cardiovascular disease, cancer and the list go on and on. It also causes a hormonal roller coaster alternating high levels of blood sugar and insulin affecting attitude and concentration (probably you have heard to avoid giving sugar to a hyperactive kid). Each time you buy a product take a look at the label and if it has a word that ends in -ose (like fructose) it means it's sugar. One single product can contain five or six types of sugar!

Artificial Sweeteners

Beyond Diet does not promote the use (or ingest) of artificial sweeteners because they will keep people craving sweets and never been able to stop carbohydrate cravings. Artificial sweeteners are selling like "healthy products", in fact they are toxic for the liver. Almost every diet or sugar-free free product as well as children snacks and flavored waters contain artificial sweeteners. Avoid any product with saccharin, aspartame and sucralose.

Stevia

Now we are talking! Stevia is a great natural alternative, it is actually an herb and it is extremely sweet (hundred times more than sugar!), it is calorie free and it's not toxic for the body. Stevia can be used to sweeten drinks, or even to bake. So here is the perfect solution if you enjoy a sweet tea.

Chocolate

Okay chocolate lovers, here are the good news: you are going to be able to enjoy a piece of chocolate every now and then; yes, healthy chocolate not the ones that have been suppress to heavy process. Not white or caramel filled chocolate, the best choice here is dark chocolate with at least a 70% of raw cacao. I know this is not what you were expecting but this is the healthy chocolate and I assure you that you will end loving it too!

Fats (for cooking)

There are a wide variety of oils available in the market but which one is the best? Well it all depends on each type of cooking according to their smoke points (you shouldn't reach this point) here is the list:

No heat fats: Fish oil, liver oil and flaxseed oil

Low heat fats: Pumpkin and sunflower oils

Medium heat fats: Olive and sesame oils

High heat fats: coconut oil and ghee

Lunch Time

People find lunch the most difficult meal during the day because it comes exactly when they are busy at work or running errands. It's so hard to take a few minutes to sit and have a healthy lunch, so in the hopes of having something "healthy" we grab some snacks instead of eating nothing at all. Consider that snacks don't have to be unhealthy; there are many nutritious snack alternatives like fruits. If you think about your typical day you can choose something easily transportable. Here we show you the snacks you shouldn't eat although you are trying to be healthy. These are "not healthy options" and if you are wishing to watch some changes in the scale you must avoid them.

1) Fat-free products: Maybe you are asking yourself "why should I avoid these products if they are fat free?" Well these kinds of products are highly processed and contain big amounts of sugar and fat replacers to keep their taste. A little bit of fat is not so bad at all!

2) Smoothies: Who doesn't love smoothies? They taste delicious and are a good option as a snack, but wait! Shops prepare smoothies with frozen yoghurt or ice cream and sugar. The good news is that you can prepare them at home in a healthy way.

3) Sushi: People often think of sushi as a good choice for a snack, besides, what's wrong with fish? It's not the fish, what's it's wrapped in is the problem. White rice and processed like cream cheese. It would be better to avoid it counting that you won't have just a roll.

4) Veggie Chips: This is a huge myth! They are fried in oil and sprinkled with lots of salt and preservatives. It doesn't matter if it is a broccoli chip; it still is a fried chip.

5) Salad dressings: Salads are great for lunch but guess what? You overload it with your favorite dressing loaded with big amounts of fat and preservatives. Goodbye to the healthy salad! Instead of adding a salad dressing to your lettuce try some vinegar, lemon and olive oil.

6) Frozen pizza, fried foods and highly processed foods: These foods are favorite of everybody but there are healthy ways to consume them, for example instead of eating spaghetti in a can you can prepare a whole grain spaghetti with natural tomato sauce. Don't buy a bag of chips; cook your own potatoes in the oven instead of frying them.

7) Flavored Yogurt or with fruit on the bottom: Don't get me wrong, you can eat yogurt, it has probiotics and protein, just eat it plain, Greek yogurt is excellent. Yogurt with fruit on the bottom in not healthy! Probably they have fructose corn syrup; of course not natural fruit is included.

8) Liquid Egg or Egg Beaters: When you buy eggbeaters or liquid eggs you may think it is fine, well guess what? These "egg alternatives" contain sweeteners or added color, besides there's no yolk in there and yolks hold a big percentage of an egg's protein.

5 Foods You Should Never Eat

1) Artificial Sweeteners: If you consume artificial sweeteners the liver gets stress and it is unable to get rid of fat. This fat will get stored in your body.

2) Margarine: Like all hydrogenated oils, margarine will cause you to store fat in your body.

3) Orange Juice: It has a big amount of sugar and simple carbohydrates.

4) Soy Products: Like sweeteners soy products give a hard time to the liver, disabling it for getting rid of fat.

5) Whole Grain Bread: The simple carbohydrates in it quickly transform into sugar, increasing blood sugar levels.

Chapter 5. Calories

How many calories enough? Enough must be the amount of calories to provide energy for your body to perform all the necessary functions but it's not the same for everyone it vary from each person and there are different facts to consider like age, weight, daily activities, sleep hours, metabolism type, etc.

The more fuel you give to your body the harder your metabolism will work and the healthier your body will be. People can eat and still maintain the ideal weight.

Sometimes eating more food means loose more weight. Let me explain how this works: The number of calories that go in does not equal the number of calories that go out. What really matters is what the body does with the food that receives. For example, if you eat a fruit, it is a whole natural food without any additives like sugar or preservatives. At the very first moment the body receives the natural food, it instantly recognizes it and know what to do with that food. It is easier for the body to digest it, then it begins to distribute nutrients improving body function and as a result of this your metabolism will increase.

On the contrary when you eat a processed food your body has no idea what to do with it. It doesn't know how to digest it or what nutrients can be used. These products are not food, they have no nutritional value and your body doesn't know how to process them, so the "fake food" ends up being stored as fat.

That's why so many people are overweight, because they are eating chemical laden foods. When chemicals enter your body, it starts to work storing fat cells while protecting vital organs, and if you eat or drink these chemicals everyday fat cells get bigger. Many products available on the market claim to be light, or 100 % natural, low fat, zero-calorie but if you take a closer look at the label you can read things like silicon dioxide, what is that? A good rule here is "If you can't read it, don't eat it". These chemicals are disguised as healthy options to lose weight when the truth is that they are the toxins clogging you digestive system causing to store more body fat. They are foods that quickly transform to sugar inside your body. Some examples of these products are cereals, muffins and granola. As a result of consuming too much sugar your metabolism will slow down and you won't lose weight so fast. Having too much blood sugar increases fat accumulation. In the other hand having too little blood sugar will cause cravings and hunger so it is important to consume the right amount of sugar to cause fat loss.

Another big enemy are simple carbs because they turn into sugar fast, whole grain breads, pastas, cereals and crackers even if they come with health claims written on the package.

Conclusion

Beyond Diet could be a bit challenging for newcomers. This program involves huge lifestyle changes. Changing your entire lifestyle and diet is not going to be easy but of course you will be rewarded for all your efforts getting a healthier and well-balanced lifestyle.

There are countless recipes you can prepare within the Beyond Diet Plan. Changing your eating habits doesn't mean that you won't enjoy food ever again.

Thank You Page

I want to personally thank you for reading my book. I hope you found information in this book useful and I would be very grateful if you could leave your honest review about this book. I certainly want to thank you in advance for doing this.

Lightning Source UK Ltd.
Milton Keynes UK
UKOW01f1925240715

255801UK00012B/184/P